EPILEPSY DIET GUIDE BOOK

A Complete Guide to the Epilepsy Diet: Dietary Approaches for Relief from Epilepsy

LARRY HERMAN

Copyright © 2024 by LARRY HERMAN

All Rights Reserved.

Table of Contents

Introduction

The Epilepsy Diet, Commonly Referred To As The Ketogenic Diet, Is A Therapeutic Dietary Strategy Utilized For Many Years To Treat Epilepsy, A Neurological Condition Marked By Recurring Seizures. This Diet Aims To Trigger Ketosis In The Body, Where It Mainly Uses Ketones, Generated From The Breakdown Of Lipids, As An Energy Source Rather Than Glucose.

The Ketogenic Diet Is Not Universally Applicable And Can Vary In Its Composition, Typically Emphasizing High Fat, Low Carbohydrate, And Moderate Protein Intake. This Distinctive Balance Of Macronutrients Is Thought To Modify The Metabolism

And Neurotransmitter Function In The Brain, Decreasing The Occurrence And Intensity Of Seizures In Certain Individuals.

Essential Elements Of The Epilepsy Diet:

• The Epilepsy Diet Is High In Good Fats Such Avocados, Nuts, Seeds, And Oils, Providing The Majority Of Calories. A High-Fat Content Is Essential For Initiating The Formation Of Ketones In The Liver.

• **Low Carbohydrate**: This Diet Restricts Carbohydrates To Reduce The Body's Dependence On Glucose. Carbohydrate-Rich Foods Like Grains,

Sweets, And Starchy Vegetables Are Restricted To A Set Daily Limit.

• **Moderate Protein:** Protein Consumption Is Controlled To Prevent Excessive Gluconeogenesis, The Conversion Of Protein Into Glucose By The Body. Protein Sources Comprise Meat, Fish, Eggs, And Dairy Products.

• The Major Objective Of The Epileptic Diet Is To Reach And Sustain A State Of Ketosis. During This Metabolic State, The Body Utilizes Fat As Fuel, Generating Ketones That Can Pass Across The Blood-Brain Barrier To Serve As An Alternate Energy Source For The Brain.

Uses of the Epilepsy Diet:

• The Ketogenic Diet Is Used As A Treatment Approach For Patients, Particularly Children, Who Have Epilepsy That Does Not Respond To Medication. Evidence Indicates That It Can Decrease The Frequency Of Seizures And Enhance Seizure Management In Certain Instances.

• Ongoing Research Is Investigating The Possible Advantages Of The Ketogenic Diet In Many Neurological Illnesses, Including Alzheimer's Disease, Parkinson's Disease, And Brain Cancers, Beyond Epilepsy.

3. Metabolic Health: The Diet Is Being Recognized For Its Possible Effects On

Metabolic Health, Weight Loss, And Insulin Sensitivity, Prompting Some To Follow It For Reasons Not Related To Epilepsy.

It Is Essential For Individuals Contemplating The Epilepsy Diet To Seek Help From Healthcare Specialists Due To The Diet's Stringent Criteria, Which May Present Difficulties In Terms Of Nutritional Sufficiency And Compliance. Regular Medical Oversight Is Crucial To Assess Its Efficacy And Address Possible Negative Effects.

CHAPTER ONE
Categories of Epilepsy

Epilepsy Is A Neurological Illness Marked By Repeated Seizures, Which Are Abrupt, Uncontrolled Electrical Disruptions In The Brain. Epilepsy Has Different Forms, Each Categorized According To The Features Of The Seizures, The Brain Regions Involved, And The Root Causes. Below Are Few Prevalent Forms Of Epilepsy:

1. Seizures Affecting the Entire Brain.

• **Absence Seizures (Petit Mal):** Short Periods Of Unconsciousness, Typically Accompanied By Slight Bodily Movements. The Individual May Seem

To Be Gazing Into The Void And Might Not Be Conscious Of The Seizure.

• Tonic-Clonic Seizures, Also Known As Grand Mal Seizures, Include Loss Of Consciousness, Bodily Stiffness (Tonic Phase), And Rhythmic Jerking And Convulsions (Clonic Phase).

• Myoclonic Seizures Are Characterized By Abrupt, Short Muscle Jerks Or Twitches That Might Impact Certain Muscles Or The Entire Body.

2. Partial Epilepsy:

• Simple Partial Seizures Impact A Distinct Region Of The Brain, Resulting In Localized Symptoms As Twitching, Tingling, Or Alterations In Emotions

Or Perception. Consciousness Remains Intact.

Complex Partial Seizures Entail A Change In Consciousness Or Awareness, Often Accompanied By Atypical Behaviors. The Individual May Experience Postictal Amnesia Following The Seizure.

3. Generalized And Focal Onset Seizures:

• Unknown Onset Seizures Refer To Seizures When It Is Uncertain Whether They Start In A Single Area Of The Brain (Focal) Or Include The Entire Brain (Generalized).

4. Seizure Spasms:

• Infantile Spasms Typically Manifest In Newborns Aged Between 3 And 12 Months. Manifesting Abrupt, Short-Lived Contractions Of Flexor Or Extensor Muscles, Frequently Occurring In Groups.

5. Lennox-Gastaut Syndrome

• Childhood Epilepsy Is A Serious Condition With Various Seizure Types, Intellectual Impairment, And Aberrant EEG Patterns.

6. Juvenile Myoclonic Epilepsy (JME):

• Usually Starts Around Puberty And Includes Myoclonic Jerks, Generalized

Tonic-Clonic Seizures, And Occasionally Absence Seizures.

7. Photosensitive Epilepsy:

• Seizures Induced By Exposure To Flickering Lights Or Visual Patterns.

8. Temporal Lobe Epilepsy

• Temporal Lobe Seizures. Commonly Linked To Complex Partial Seizures And May Include Changes In Awareness, Memory, And Feelings.

9. Frontal Lobe Epilepsy:

• Frontal Lobe Seizures Are Seizures That Start In The Frontal Lobes And Are Typically Marked By Motor Movements, Abnormal Behaviors, And Changes In Awareness.

10. Seizures Originating In The Occipital Lobe Of The Brain.

• Seizures Originating In The Occipital Lobes Can Impact Vision And Can Lead To Visual Hallucinations.

Epilepsy Is A Varied Disorder, And Individuals May Have Varying Experiences With Seizures. The Taxonomy And Language Of Epilepsy Types May Change As Our Knowledge Of The Illness Progresses. Accurate Diagnosis And Proper Treatment Are Essential For Patients With Epilepsy, And A Healthcare Provider, Typically A Neurologist, Is Vital In Overseeing The Management Of The Illness.

Diet's Impact on Epilepsy Management

Diet Is Crucial In Managing Epilepsy, Especially For Persons With Drug-Resistant Epilepsy Or Those Exploring Alternative Therapy Alternatives. The Primary Dietary Strategy For Managing Epilepsy Is The Ketogenic Diet. Here Is A Summary Of The Function Of Nutrition In Managing Epilepsy:

1. Ketogenic Diet:

• The Ketogenic Diet Is A Dietary Regimen Characterized By High Fat, Low Carbohydrate, And Moderate Protein Intake. Its Goal Is To Trigger Ketosis, A Metabolic State In Which The Body Predominantly Relies On

Ketones For Energy Rather Than Glucose.

• Ketones Are Generated During The Breakdown Of Fats In The Body And Have The Ability To Pass Through The Blood-Brain Barrier, Offering An Alternative Energy Source For The Brain.

• The Ketogenic Diet Has Proven To Be Useful, Particularly In Children With Drug-Resistant Epilepsy, In Decreasing Seizure Frequency And Enhancing Seizure Control.

Various Forms Of The Ketogenic Diet Exist, Such As The Conventional Ketogenic Diet, The Modified Atkins Diet, The Medium-Chain Triglyceride

(MCT) Diet, And The Low Glycemic Index Treatment (LGIT), Providing Options For Food Selection And Macronutrient Proportions.

2. Modified Atkins Diet

• The Modified Atkins Diet Is A Less Rigorous Version Of The Ketogenic Diet That Permits Higher Protein And Carbohydrate Consumption While Still Encouraging Ketosis.

• Medical Adherence (MAD) Has Shown Efficacy In Decreasing Seizure Frequency And Enhancing Seizure Management, Especially In Adults And Teenagers With Epilepsy.

3. Low Glycemic Index Treatment (LGIT):

• LGIT Emphasizes The Use Of Carbohydrates With A Low Glycemic Index To Reduce Blood Sugar Fluctuations And Support Ketosis.

• LGIT Has Proven To Be Advantageous For Persons With Epilepsy, Particularly Those Who Find It Challenging To Adhere To The Stringent Carbohydrate Limitations Of Other Ketogenic Diets.

4. Medium-Chain Triglyceride (MCT) Diet:

• The MCT Diet Includes MCT Oil, Which Is More Easily Turned Into

Ketones Than Long-Chain Fatty Acids Found In Regular Dietary Fats.

• MCT Oil Is Commonly Included In Meals To Enhance The Production Of Ketones And Sustain Ketosis.

5. Gluten-Free and Casein-Free (GFCF) Diet:

• Some People With Epilepsy, Especially Those With Other Conditions Like Autism Spectrum Disorder, May Find Relief From A Gluten-Free And Casein-Free Diet Due To Potential Food Sensitivities That Could Worsen Seizure Activity.

6. Personalized Strategies:

• It Is Crucial To Recognize That The Efficacy Of Dietary Treatments For

Epilepsy Might Differ Among Individuals, And Not Everyone May Have A Satisfactory Response.

•   Healthcare Experts, Especially Neurologists And Dietitians With Expertise In Epilepsy Management, Are Essential In Customizing Dietary Interventions For Individuals, Tracking Their Development, And Ensuring Nutritional Sufficiency.

Dietary Therapies, Such As The Ketogenic Diet And Its Modifications, Show Promise For Managing Epilepsy, Particularly For Those Who Do Not Respond Well To Standard Antiepileptic Drugs Or Who Suffer From Notable Adverse Effects. Individuals Interested In Using Dietary

Therapy For Epilepsy Should Do So Under Medical Supervision To Guarantee Safety, Effectiveness, And Nutritional Adequacy.

CHAPTER TWO
Principles Of The Epilepsy Diet

The Epilepsy Diet, Including The Ketogenic Diet And Its Modifications, Is Based On Specific Dietary Concepts Designed To Trigger And Sustain A State Of Ketosis. The Fundamental Components Of The Epilepsy Diet Are As Follows:

1. Excessive Consumption Of Fats:

• The Main Principle Of The Epilepsy Diet Is A Substantial Rise In The Intake Of Dietary Fats. Fats Are The Main Energy Source For The Body And Play A Vital Role In Ketone Synthesis.

• Healthy Fats Including Avocados, Nuts, Seeds, Olive Oil, And Fatty

Seafood Are Highlighted For Achieving The Proper Balance Of Macronutrients.

2. Reduced Consumption Of Carbohydrates:

• Carbohydrate Consumption Is Restricted To Trigger And Sustain Ketosis. Limiting Carbohydrates Decreases Glucose Availability, Prompting The Body To Use Fats For Energy.

• Foods Rich In Carbs, Such As Sweets, Grains, And Starchy Vegetables, Are Reduced Or Removed.

3. Moderate Protein Intake:

• Protein Consumption Is Regulated To Avoid Excessive Gluconeogenesis,

Which Is The Conversion Of Protein Into Glucose By The Body. Excessive Protein Intake Can Disrupt The Process Of Ketosis.

• Protein Foods Like Meat, Fish, Eggs, And Dairy Are Consumed In Moderation.

4. Therapeutic Objective:

• The Basic Goal Of The Epileptic Diet Is To Reach And Sustain A State Of Ketosis. During Ketosis, The Body Generates Ketones By Breaking Down Fats, Which Then Act As A Substitute Energy Source For The Brain.

• Ketosis Is Usually Verified By Testing For Ketones In Urine, Blood, Or Breath.

5. Personalized Strategies:

• The Epilepsy Diet Is Not Universally Applicable. It Necessitates Customized Modifications Depending On Aspects Like Age, Weight, Underlying Health Issues, And Personal Preferences.

• Various Forms Of The Ketogenic Diet, Including The Standard Ketogenic Diet, Modified Atkins Diet, Medium-Chain Triglyceride (MCT) Diet, And Low Glycemic Index Therapy (LGIT), Provide Adaptability To Suit Different Requirements And Choices.

6. Medical Oversight and Surveillance:

• Initiating And Adhering To The Epilepsy Diet Should Be Supervised By

Healthcare Specialists, Such As Neurologists And Dietitians With Expertise In Epilepsy Care.

• Regularly Monitoring Ketone Levels, Seizure Frequency, And General Nutritional Condition Is Essential To Evaluate The Diet's Success And Make Any Needed Changes.

7. Adherence and Lifestyle Factors:

• Following The Epilepsy Diet Can Be Difficult, And One Should Consider Lifestyle Aspects Like Social And Cultural Influences.

• Support From Healthcare Professionals, Together With Education And Resources For Patients And Their Families, Is Crucial For

Successful Implementation And Sustained Adherence In The Long Term.

8. Possible Adverse Reactions:

• The Ketogenic Diet For Epilepsy Can Lead To Adverse Effects Such As Constipation, Gastrointestinal Discomfort, And Vitamin Shortages. Proper Supplementation And Monitoring Are Crucial To Deal With Such Problems.

The Epilepsy Diet Is Based On Carefully Balancing Macronutrients To Achieve And Sustain Ketosis, Which Helps In Treating Epilepsy For Therapeutic Purposes. Personalized Care, Medical Oversight, And

Continuous Assistance Are Essential Elements To Guarantee The Safety And Efficacy Of The Diet For Individuals With Epilepsy.

Epilepsy Diet Overview

An Overview Of The Epilepsy Diet Focuses On The Ketogenic Diet And Its Modifications, Which Are Dietary Strategies Aimed At Managing Epilepsy, Especially In Instances Of Drug-Resistant Seizures. The Essential Components Of The Epilepsy Diet Are As Follows:

1. Ketogenic Diet (KD):

• The Ketogenic Diet Is A Dietary Approach Characterized By High Fat Intake, Low Carbohydrate

Consumption, And Moderate Protein Intake With The Goal Of Achieving And Sustaining A State Of Ketosis In The Body.

• Ketosis Is A Metabolic Condition Where The Body Predominantly Utilizes Ketones, Derived From The Breakdown Of Lipids, As A Substitute Energy Source For The Brain Rather Than Glucose.

The Traditional Ketogenic Diet Usually Consists Of A Ratio Of Fats To The Total Of Proteins And Carbs Of 3:1 Or 4:1, Equating To Three Or Four Grams Of Fat For Each Gram Of Protein And Carbohydrate Combined.

2. Modified Atkins Diet

• The Modified Atkins Diet Is A Version Of The Ketogenic Diet That Permits Increased Protein And Carbohydrate Consumption While Maintaining Ketosis.

• The Modified Ketogenic Diet Is Less Rigorous Than The Traditional Ketogenic Diet And May Be Better Suited For Teenagers And Adults.

3. Medium-Chain Triglyceride (MCT) Diet:

• The MCT Diet Includes Medium-Chain Triglyceride Oil, A Fat That Is Turned Into Ketones Faster Than Long-Chain Fats.

• MCT Oil Is Commonly Used As A Dietary Supplement To Offer A Conveniently Available Source Of Ketones.

4. Low Glycemic Index Treatment (LGIT):

• LGIT Emphasizes The Consumption Of Carbohydrates With A Low Glycemic Index To Support Stable Blood Sugar Levels And Encourage Ketosis.

It Permits A Higher Consumption Of Carbs Than Other Ketogenic Diets.

5. Commencement and Sustenance:

• Starting The Epilepsy Diet Often Includes A Slow Transition, With Careful Monitoring Of Ketone Levels

And Changes Made To Reach The Intended Therapeutic Outcome.

• Once Ketosis Is Reached, It Is Crucial To Maintain The Diet By Continuously Monitoring, Making Adjustments, And Receiving Regular Medical Supervision.

6. Efficiency in Seizure Control:

• The Epilepsy Diet, Specifically The Ketogenic Diet, Has Proven To Be Beneficial In Decreasing Seizure Frequency And Enhancing Seizure Management In Certain Individuals, Notably Those With Drug-Resistant Epilepsy.

• The Mechanism Of Action Is Not Completely Understood, However It Is

Thought To Entail Changes In Brain Metabolism And Neurotransmitter Function.

7. Factors to Take Into Account and Difficulties:

• Following The Epilepsy Diet Can Be Difficult Because It Is Quite Restricted And May Lead To Adverse Effects Like Constipation, Gastrointestinal Discomfort, And Vitamin Shortages.

It Is Essential For Patients To Acquire Instruction And Help From Healthcare Professionals Such As Neurologists And Dietitians To Overcome Obstacles And Maintain Adequate Nutritional Balance.

8. Possible Applications Other Than Epilepsy:

• Research Is Currently Being Conducted To Investigate The Possible Advantages Of Ketogenic Diets In Many Neurological Illnesses And Metabolic Problems, Including Alzheimer's Disease, Parkinson's Disease, And Obesity.

Overall, The Epilepsy Diet, Namely The Ketogenic Diet And Its Modifications, Is A Treatment Method That Involves Adjusting Macronutrient Consumption To Trigger Ketosis And Control Epilepsy. Its Efficacy, Personalized Approach, And Possible Uses Outside Of Epilepsy Make It A Topic Of Further Investigation And Medical Attention.

Categories of Epilepsy Diets

Various Epilepsy Diets Exist, Each With A Distinct Nutritional Composition And Strategy For Controlling Seizures. These Diets Are Commonly Recommended For Patients With Epilepsy, Especially Those Who Have Not Had Success With Conventional Antiepileptic Drugs. Below Are Some Primary Categories Of Epilepsy Diets:

1. Ketogenic Diet (KD):

• The Ketogenic Diet Is A Dietary Approach That Is High In Fat, Low In Carbohydrates, And Moderate In Protein. Its Purpose Is To Trigger Ketosis, A Metabolic Condition In Which The Body Predominantly

Utilizes Ketones For Energy Rather Than Glucose.

• The Traditional Ketogenic Diet Usually Offers A Ratio Of Fats To The Combined Proteins And Carbs Of 3:1 Or 4:1.

• Variants Of The Ketogenic Diet Comprise The Modified Atkins Diet (MAD), Medium-Chain Triglyceride (MCT) Diet, And Low Glycemic Index Treatment (LGIT).

2. Modified Atkins Diet:

• The Modified Atkins Diet (MAD) Is A Less Rigorous Version Of The Ketogenic Diet That Permits Increased Consumption Of Protein And

Carbohydrates While Still Encouraging The Body To Enter A State Of Ketosis.

It Is Commonly Utilized In Teens And Adults And May Be More Practical For Long-Term Compliance.

3. Medium-Chain Triglyceride (MCT) Diet:

• The MCT Diet Includes Medium-Chain Triglyceride Oil, Which Is Rapidly Turned Into Ketones Compared To Long-Chain Lipids.

• MCT Oil Is Frequently Used In Meals To Enhance Ketone Generation And Sustain Ketosis.

4. Low Glycemic Index Treatment (LGIT):

• LGIT Emphasizes The Use Of Carbohydrates With A Low Glycemic Index To Stabilize Blood Sugar Levels And Sustain Ketosis.

It Permits A Higher Consumption Of Carbs In Comparison To Other Ketogenic Diets.

5. Atkins Diet:

• The Atkins Diet, Especially The Induction Phase, Has Similarities With The Ketogenic Diet, But It Is Not Expressly Intended For Epilepsy. It Entails Consuming A Reduced Amount Of Carbohydrates, Which Results In

The Body Entering A Condition Of Ketosis.

6. Paleolithic Diet (Paleo):

• The Paleo Diet Focuses On Eating Foods That Were Accessible During The Paleolithic Era, With An Emphasis On Lean Meats, Seafood, Fruits, Vegetables, Nuts, And Seeds.

• Some People With Epilepsy May Experience Advantages From Following A Paleo Diet, Albeit There Is Insufficient Data On Its Effectiveness.

7. Gluten-Free and Casein-Free (GFCF) Diet:

• Some People With Epilepsy, Especially Those With Other Conditions Like Autism Spectrum

Disorder, May Adhere To A GFCF Diet, Which Involves Avoiding Gluten-Containing Grains And Dairy Products.

8. Adapted Ketogenic Diet For Targeted Conditions:

• Specific Modified Ketogenic Diets Are Customized To Target The Metabolic Problems Associated With Certain Conditions Like Glucose Transporter Type 1 Deficiency Syndrome (GLUT1 DS).

The Efficacy Of These Diets Can Differ From Person To Person, And The Selection Of A Diet May Be Influenced By Factors Like Age, Medical Background, And Lifestyle. Dietary Therapies For Epilepsy Should Be

Supervised By Healthcare Specialists Such As Neurologists And Dietitians To Guarantee Correct Execution, Supervision, And Nutritional Sufficiency. Individuals' Reactions To These Diets Vary, And Modifications May Be Required As Time Goes On.

CHAPTER THREE
Understanding The Mechanisms Of The Epilepsy Diet

The Epilepsy Diet, Namely The Ketogenic Diet And Its Modifications, Functions By Initiating And Sustaining A State Of Ketosis In The Body. Ketosis Is A Metabolic Condition When The Body Predominantly Uses Ketones, Derived From The Breakdown Of Lipids, As Its Main Energy Source Rather Than Depending On Glucose. The Precise Mechanisms By Which The Epilepsy Diet Produces Its Therapeutic Effects Are Not Completely Understood, However Several Crucial Aspects Contribute To Its Effectiveness In Controlling Seizures:

1. Metabolic Changes:

• The High-Fat, Low-Carbohydrate Nature Of The Epilepsy Diet Causes A Notable Change In The Body's Metabolism. When Carbs Are Limited, The Body Enhances The Breakdown Of Lipids To Generate Ketones Due To Decreased Glucose Availability.

• Ketones, Such As Beta-Hydroxybutyrate, Acetoacetate, And Acetone, Become The Main Source Of Energy For The Brain In Ketosis.

2. Neural Excitability Stabilization:

• Ketones Are Proposed To Stabilize Neuronal Excitability. This Could Be Due To Alterations In Ion Channel

Activity And Neurotransmitter Secretion In The Brain.

The Decreased Presence Of Glucose, Which Can Lead To Heightened Brain Activity, Can Possibly Be Involved In Managing Seizures.

3. Modulation of Neurotransmitters:

• The Epilepsy Diet Can Impact The Amount And Function Of Neurotransmitters In The Brain, Including Gamma-Aminobutyric Acid (GABA) And Glutamate.

• GABA Is An Inhibitory Neurotransmitter That Regulates Neuronal Excitability, Whereas Glutamate Is An Excitatory Neurotransmitter. Adjusting The

Equilibrium Of These Neurotransmitters Could Help Manage Seizures.

4. Anti-Inflammatory Properties:

• Some Research Indicates That The Ketogenic Diet Might Possess Anti-Inflammatory Qualities, Perhaps Enhancing Its Ability To Protect The Nervous System.

• Inflammation In The Brain Is Linked To The Onset And Reappearance Of Seizures, And Decreasing Inflammation Could Be Advantageous For Managing Seizures.

5. Improved Mitochondrial Function:

• Ketones Are Utilized More Efficiently By Mitochondria, The Cellular Energy-Producing Organelles, In Comparison To Glucose. Improved Mitochondrial Function Could Benefit Cellular Health, Including Brain Cells.

• Enhanced Mitochondrial Function May Play A Role In The Neuroprotective Benefits Seen In Those Who Adhere To The Epileptic Diet.

6. Epigenetic Alterations:

• The Epilepsy Diet Can Cause Epigenetic Alterations That Impact

The Activity Of Genes Related To Brain Function And Metabolism.

• The Alterations May Contribute To The Diet's Lasting Therapeutic Impact On Seizure Management.

Variability In Response To The Epilepsy Diet Exists Among Individuals, And Not All Epilepsy Patients Will Derive The Same Degree Of Improvement. The Diet Is Usually Recommended For Those With Drug-Resistant Epilepsy Or Those Who Suffer From Intolerable Side Effects From Drugs. Medical Oversight, Consistent Observation, And Modifications To The Diet Are Essential To Guarantee Safety, Effectiveness, And Nutritional

Sufficiency. Consult Healthcare Specialists, Such As Neurologists And Dietitians, Before Deciding To Start The Epilepsy Diet.

Beginning The Epilepsy Diet

Initiating The Epilepsy Diet, Specifically The Ketogenic Diet, Requires Meticulous Preparation, Collaboration With Healthcare Providers, And A Gradual Shift To The New Dietary Regimen. Here Are Methods To Initiate The Epilepsy Diet For Patients Or Caregivers:

1. Meeting With Medical Professionals:

• Prior To Beginning The Epileptic Diet, Seek Guidance From A

Healthcare Team Specializing In Epilepsy Management. This May Involve A Neurologist, Dietician, And Other Pertinent Professionals.

• The Healthcare Team Will Evaluate The Individual's Medical History, Current Medications, And Specific Dietary Requirements To Decide If The Epilepsy Diet Is Appropriate.

2. Learning Materials:

• Explore The Epilepsy Diet And Its Several Forms By Utilizing Educational Materials Offered By Healthcare Professionals, Reliable Websites, And Epilepsy Groups.

• Understanding The Diet's Principles, Potential Obstacles, And Monitoring

Requirements Is Essential For Successful Adoption.

3. Select The Appropriate Diet Type:

• Collaborate With Healthcare Providers To Identify The Best Appropriate Epilepsy Diet Considering Individual Aspects Including Age, Lifestyle, And Preferences.

• Possible Options Are The Standard Ketogenic Diet, Modified Atkins Diet (MAD), Medium-Chain Triglyceride (MCT) Diet, Or Low Glycemic Index Treatment (LGIT).

4. Planning Meals:

• Create A Meal Plan With The Prescribed Macronutrient Ratios For The Selected Epilepsy Diet.

Focus On Incorporating Healthy Fats, Consuming Moderate Amounts Of Protein, And Choosing Low-Carbohydrate Foods. Incorporate A Diverse Range Of Foods To Guarantee A Balanced And Nutritionally Sufficient Diet.

5. Gradual Change:

• Gradually Introduce The Epilepsy Diet To Reduce Negative Effects And Aid In The Individual's Adjustment To The New Eating Regimen.

• Gradually Decreasing Carbohydrate Intake Over A Span Of Days Or Weeks May Be Advised.

6. Surveillance And Ketone Analysis:

• Regularly Monitor Ketone Levels By Urine, Blood, Or Breath Ketone Testing Methods. This Helps To Guarantee That The Body Is In A State Of Ketosis.

Healthcare Specialists Will Provide Guidance On Conducting Ketone Testing And Understanding The Outcomes.

7. Hydration And Electrolyte Equilibrium:

• Proper Hydration Is Essential, And Those On The Epilepsy Diet Should Monitor Their Electrolyte Levels.

Increased Water Consumption And Suitable Electrolyte Supplementation May Be Required.

8. Dealing with Obstacles and Adverse Reactions:

• Be Ready For Any Hurdles Like Adherence Issues, Stomach Pain, Or Vitamin Deficits.

Collaborate With Healthcare Specialists To Manage Side Effects And Modify The Diet As Needed.

9. Regular Monitoring:

• Arrange Periodic Follow-Up Meetings With The Healthcare Team To Track Advancements, Modify The Diet As Necessary, And Discuss Any Issues.

Continued Support Is Crucial For Maintaining Adherence Over The Long Run.

10. Lifestyle Factors:

• Consider How The Epilepsy Diet Aligns With The Individual's Lifestyle, Taking Into Account Social, Cultural, And Practical Factors.

• Prepare In Advance For Social Gatherings, Trips, And Other Occasions To Ensure You Stick To Your Dietary Requirements.

Implementing The Epilepsy Diet Necessitates Careful Consideration And Continuous Help From Healthcare Specialists. It Is Advised Not To Begin The Diet Without Medical Oversight,

Particularly For Persons With Preexisting Health Issues Or Those On Medication. The Healthcare Team Will Assist The Individual In Navigating The Procedure, Prioritizing Safety And Maximizing The Possible Advantages Of The Diet For Managing Epilepsy.

CHAPTER FOUR
Foods To Include In The Epilepsy Diet

The Epilepsy Diet, Particularly The Ketogenic Diet And Its Variations, Involves Specific Food Choices To Achieve The Desired Macronutrient Ratios And Induce Ketosis. Here Are Examples Of Foods That Are Typically Included In The Epilepsy Diet:

1. Healthy Fats: MCT Oil (Medium-Chain Triglycerides) , Avocados ,Olive Oil ,Coconut Oil

• Nuts And Seeds (Such As Flaxseeds, Chia Seeds, Walnuts, And Almonds), Butter And Ghee

2. Sources of Protein: Meat (Such As Hog, Lamb, Chicken, and Beef)

Fish and Shellfish

Eggs

• Dairy Products (Such As Full-Fat Yogurt and Cheese)

• Tempeh and Tofu

3. Low-Carbohydrate Vegetables: Cruciferous Vegetables (Such As Broccoli, Cauliflower, and Brussels Sprouts)

• Leafy Greens (Such As Spinach, Kale, And Lettuce)

• Zucchini

• Bell Peppers

• Cabbage

• Asparagus

4. Berries (In Moderation):

- Berries With Less Carbs, Like Raspberries, Strawberries, And Blueberries, Can Be Included In Moderation.

5. Herbs and Spices:

- Herbs (Like Basil, Cilantro, Mint, Oregano)
- Spices (Like Turmeric, Cumin, Cinnamon, Ginger)
- These Enhance The Flavor Of Food Without Adding A Substantial Amount Of Carbohydrates.

6. Low-Glycemic Fruits (In Moderation): Because They Have Fewer Carbohydrates Than Other

Fruits, Fruits Including Avocados, Tomatoes, And Some Berries Can Be Consumed In Moderation.

7. Full-Fat Dairy (In Moderation):

• Since They Are A Source Of Both Fat And Protein, Full-Fat Dairy Products Like Cheese And Yogurt Can Be Consumed In Moderation.

8. Beverages:

• The Main Beverage And Essential For Maintaining Hydration Is Water.

• Black Coffee (Without Additional Sugar) And Herbal Teas (Without Sweetness) Are Usually OK.

9. Sweeteners (In Moderation): You Can Add Sweetness Without

Dramatically Raising Your Blood Sugar Levels By Using Non-Nutritive Sweeteners Like Erythritol Or Stevia In Moderation.

10. Nutrient-Dense Foods: Include Nutrient-Dense Foods In Your Diet To Make Sure You're Getting Enough Vitamins And Minerals. This Could Include Leafy Greens, A Range Of Vibrant Veggies, And Organ Meats.

It's Important To Note That Portion Sizes And Overall Macronutrient Ratios Vary Depending On The Specific Type Of Epilepsy Diet Being Followed (E.G., Classic Ketogenic Diet, Modified Atkins Diet, MCT Diet). Additionally, Individual Tolerances And Responses To Certain Foods May Vary, So

Adjustments May Be Necessary Based On Personal Health Considerations And Responses To The Diet.

It Is Recommended To Work Closely With Healthcare Professionals, Including A Neurologist And A Registered Dietitian Specializing In Epilepsy Management, To Tailor The Diet To Individual Needs, Monitor Progress, And Address Any Potential Challenges Or Side Effects.

Items to Steer Clear of on an Epilepsy Diet

Certain Items Must Be Avoided In The Epileptic Diet In Order To Preserve The Precise Macronutrient Ratios Needed To Produce And Maintain Ketosis, Particularly In Ketogenic And

Related Varieties. The Following Foods Are Usually Limited Or Avoided In An Epilepsy Diet:

1. Foods High In Carbohydrates:

- Cereals and Grains, Such As Wheat, Rice, And Oats
- Bread And More Baked Items
- Pasta
- Starchy Veggies, Such As Potatoes
- Legumes (Such As Lentils And Beans)

2. Sweeteners And Sugar-Coated Foods:

- Sugar And Foods High In Sugar
- Honey, Maple Syrup, And More Sugar Substitutes

- Hydrogenated Corn Syrup

- Normal Sodas And Drinks With Added Sweetness

3. Prepared Foods:

• Sugars And Carbs That Are Concealed Are Present In Many Processed Foods. It's Crucial To Thoroughly Read Labels.

• Chips, Crackers, And Other Processed Foods Frequently Have High Carb Counts.

4. High-Glycemic Fruits:

• Fruits Heavy In Sugar, Like Bananas, Grapes, And Tropical Fruits, Should Usually Be Consumed In Moderation Or Avoided.

- Concentrated Sugars Are Also Abundant In Fruit Juices And Dried Fruits.

5. High-Glycemic Vegetables:

- Carrots And Sweet Potatoes, Two Root Vegetables That Have A Greater Carbohydrate Content, Are Off Limits.

- Take Care When Handling Tomatoes And Onions Because They Have Modest Carbohydrate Content.

6. Meats Processed and Sugar-Added:

- It's Important To Select Unprocessed And Sugar-Free Choices Because Certain Processed Meats May Have Extra Sugars.

• Examine The Labels Of Bacon, Sausages, And Cured Meats.

7. Low-Sat Content Dairy Products:

• Low-Fat Or Reduced-Fat Dairy Products May Be Prohibited In Some Epilepsy Diet Variations Due To Their Potential Greater Carbohydrate Content.

• Due To Its Increased Fat Content, Full-Fat Dairy Is Frequently Favored.

8. Spirits:

• Alcoholic Drinks Are Typically Prohibited, Particularly Those With A High Sugar Content Or Mixers.

- Alcohol May Interfere With Medication Interactions And Alter The Metabolism Of Ketone Bodies.

9. High-Glycemic Relatives:

- Restrict Your Intake Of Condiments Containing Added Sugars, Such As Ketchup And Barbecue Sauce.

- Commercial Salad Dressings Should Be Used With Caution As They Could Include Added Sugars.

10. Certain Nuts And Seeds High In Carbohydrates:

- The Epilepsy Diet Typically Includes Nuts And Seeds, But Some—Like Cashews And Chestnuts—Have Higher Carb Counts And Should Only Be Eaten In Moderation.

It's Crucial To Stress That The Precise Foods To Avoid Can Change Based On Personal Tolerances And The Kind Of Epilepsy Diet Being Followed (E.G., The Standard Ketogenic Diet, The Modified Atkins Diet, Or The MCT Diet). Close Collaboration With Medical Specialists, Such As A Neurologist And A Qualified Dietitian With Expertise In Managing Epilepsy, Guarantees Appropriate Direction, Supervision, And Diet Modifications Depending On Personal Requirements And Reactions. Sustained Support And Routine Follow-Up Meetings Are Essential For Successful Epilepsy Diet Compliance.

CHAPTER FIVE
Handling Possible Adverse Effects

Adopting An Epilepsy Diet, Particularly The Ketogenic Diet And Its Derivatives, May Result In Unintended Consequences. It's Critical To Recognize These Possible Negative Impacts And Take The Necessary Action To Mitigate Them. The Following List Of Typical Side Effects And Coping Mechanisms:

1. Keto Flu:

• Symptoms Include Headache, Nausea, Dizziness, And Irritability.

• **Approach:** A Gradual Diet Introduction, Appropriate Rest, Electrolyte Supplementation (Salt,

Potassium, And Magnesium), And Proper Hydration Can All Help Reduce Symptoms.

2. Problems With The Digestive System:

• **Symptoms:** Upset Stomach, Diarrhea, And Constipation.

• **Approach:** To Control Digestive Issues, Make Sure You Consume Enough Fiber From Low-Carb Veggies, Think About Taking Fiber Supplements, Remain Hydrated, And Modify Your Fat Intake.

3. Dehydration:

• Symptoms Include Dry Mouth, Black Urine, And Increased Thirst.

- **Approach:** Make Sure You Are Adequately Hydrated By Drinking Water Throughout The Day. Supplementing With Electrolytes Can Also Be Beneficial.

4. Inadequacies in Nutrients:

- **Symptoms:** Inadequate Intake Of Some Vitamins And Minerals As A Result Of Dietary Limitations.

- Plan A Nutritionally Balanced Diet, Discuss Supplementation If Needed, And Use Blood Tests To Track Your Body's Nutrient Levels In Collaboration With A Trained Dietitian.

5. Low Blood Sugar, Or Hypoglycemia:

- **Symptoms:** Disorientation, Weakness, and Shakiness.

- **Strategy:** To Prevent Blood Sugar Dips, Make Sure You Eat Regularly And In A Balanced Manner. You Should Also Try To Avoid Going For Extended Periods Of Time Without Eating.

6. Levels of Cholesterol:

- **Symptoms:** Increased Cholesterol, Particularly As A Result Of The Diet's High Fat Content.

- **Approach:** Consistent Lipid Profile Monitoring, Together With Expert Guidance To Evaluate And Treat Cholesterol Levels As Needed.

7. Variations in Weight:

- **Symptoms:** Unintentional Weight Gain or Loss.

- **Plan:** Continue To Track Weight, Make Necessary Calorie Adjustments, And Seek Advice From Medical Authorities.

8. Gastrointestinal Disturbance

- **Symptoms:** Bloating, Vomiting, And Nausea.

- **Approach:** Modifying The Kinds And Quantities Of Lipids Ingested, Being Well Hydrated, And Gradually Introducing The Diet Can All Help Control Gastrointestinal Discomfort.

9. Having Trouble Following the Diet:

• **Symptoms:** Difficulties Sticking To A Diet Plan Because Of Social Circumstances, Lifestyle Choices, Or Other Considerations.

• **Approach:** Seek Advice From Medical Specialists, Think About Seeing A Nutritionist, And Investigate Methods For Handling The Diet In Diverse Social And Lifestyle Settings.

10. Effect on the Mind:

• **Symptoms:** Feelings of Loneliness, Frustration, or Mood Swings.

• **Strategy:** Receiving Emotional Support From Mental Health Specialists, Support Groups, Or

Medical Professionals Might Be Helpful. For The Psychological Effects Of Dietary Modifications To Be Addressed, Open Contact With The Medical Team Is Essential.

It's Critical To Be Open And Honest About Any Adverse Effects Or Difficulties Encountered Throughout The Epilepsy Diet With Medical Specialists, Such As Neurologists And Dietitians. The Nutritional Modifications, Monitoring, And Routine Follow-Up Appointments Are All Components Of The Continuous Care And Assistance That The Medical Staff Offers. Tailored Approaches Can Be Devised To Effectively Handle Adverse Reactions And Maximize The

Nutritional Advantages In The Therapy Of Epilepsy.

Epilepsy Nutrition Plans For Various Age Groups

Depending On The Person's Age Group, Different Approaches To The Epilepsy Diet—In Particular, The Ketogenic Diet And Its Variants—May Be Taken. Below Is A Broad Summary Of Things To Think About Based On Age Groups:

1. Young Children and Adults:

• **Dietary Approach:** The Traditional Ketogenic Diet Is Frequently Adjusted For Young Children To Include A Higher Fat To Protein And Carbohydrate Ratio. The Traditional

Ketogenic Diet For Infants (CKDI) Is Another Name For This.

• **Formulae:** For Infants Who Are Not Yet Consuming Solid Foods, Ketogenic Formulae May Be Taken Into Consideration. These Mixes Are Made To Supply The Fat And Nutrients Required To Enter Ketosis.

2. Youngsters (Ages 2-12):

• Dietary Approach: In This Age Range, The Traditional Ketogenic Diet Is Frequently Employed. However, Because They Are Less Restrictive And Could Be Simpler To Follow, The Low Glycemic Index Treatment (LGIT) Or The Modified Atkins Diet (MAD) Might Be Better Suited For Some Kids.

• **Food Choices:** It's Critical To Take Into Account A Child's Capacity To Follow A Diet, As Well As Their Choices For Food, School, And Social Activities. It Is Possible To Modify The Diet To Suit The Child's Lifestyle.

3. Teenagers (Ages 13–18):

• Dietary Approach: Because Of Puberty And Growth Spurts, Adolescents May Require Different Nutrition. The Modified Atkins Diet (MAD) Or Other Less Stringent Versions That Permit Higher Intakes Of Carbohydrates And Protein Might Be Appropriate.

• **Independence And Social Factors:** Teenagers May Want Greater Control

Over How They Eat. It Is Imperative To Communicate With Healthcare Providers, Monitor Patients Often, And Provide Education On Food Choices. Social Aspects Like Interactions With Peers And School Activities Should Also Be Taken Into Account.

4. Adults:

• **Dietary Approach:** The Modified Atkins Diet (MAD) Or Other Long-Term, More Sustainable Diets May Be Beneficial For Adults With Epilepsy. Adherence To The Diet Depends On Customizing It To Each Person's Preferences And Lifestyle.

• **Health Issues**: It's Important To Take Into Account Any Coexisting

Medical Issues, Such As Metabolic Diseases Or Cardiovascular Risk Factors. It Could Be Advised To Regularly Check Cholesterol Levels And Other Health Indicators.

5. Seniors (Those Above 65):

• Dietary Approach: Seniors' Dietary Requirements And Health Conditions May Be Accommodated By Tailoring The Ketogenic Diet. Dietitians Need To Take Into Account Things Such Possible Tooth Problems, Stomach Problems, And Drug Interactions.

• **Nutrient Intake:** Seniors May Need To Consume A Certain Amount Of Protein In Order To Maintain Healthy

Muscles And Bones. Drinking Enough Water Is Also Essential.

It's Crucial To Remember That Selecting An Epilepsy Diet And Its Modifications Should Be Done After Consulting Medical Experts, Such As Neurologists And Qualified Dietitians With Experience Managing Epilepsy. The Strategy Will Be Tailored Depending On Variables Including Age, Health, Way Of Life, And Personal Preferences. Appointments For Follow-Up And Regular Monitoring Are Crucial For Determining Whether The Diet Is Working And For Making Any Necessary Modifications.

The Effects of Exercise On Epilepsy

On Epilepsy, Exercise Can Have Both Beneficial And Complicated Consequences. While Regular Exercise Is Generally Linked To A Number Of Health Advantages, Such As Enhanced Mood, Cardiovascular Health, And General Well-Being, Its Effects On Epilepsy May Differ From Person To Person. Here Are Some Important Things To Think About:

1. Possible Advantages Of Physical Activity:

• **General Health:** Exercise On A Regular Basis Improves General Health And Can Help Control Diseases Like Obesity, Diabetes, And

Cardiovascular Disease, Which May Be Linked To Epilepsy Or Have An Impact On How It Is Managed.

• **Mood And Stress:** It Is Well Recognized That Exercise Can Elevate Mood And Lower Stress Levels, Both Of Which Can Impact Seizure Activity. Reducing Stress May Be Especially Important For People Who Experience Seizures When Under Stress.

• **Cognitive Function:** Research Has Shown That Exercise Improves Memory And Attention, Two Cognitive Functions That May Be Helpful For People Who Have Epilepsy.

2. Taking Into Account People Who Have Epilepsy:

• **Individual Variability:** The Impact Of Exercise On Seizures Can Vary Among Individuals. While Some People May Experience Improvements, Others Might Notice No Significant Changes Or, In Rare Cases, An Increase In Seizure Frequency.

• **Seizure Triggers:** Exercise-Related Factors Such As Fatigue, Dehydration, Or Overheating Can Potentially Act As Triggers For Seizures In Some Individuals. Staying Hydrated And Avoiding Excessive Fatigue Is Important.

• **Types Of Exercise:** Different Types Of Exercise May Have Different Effects. Aerobic Exercise, Strength Training, And Activities Like Yoga May Be Considered, And The Choice May Depend On Individual Preferences And Limitations.

3. Precautions and Guidelines:

• **Consultation With Healthcare Professionals:** Individuals With Epilepsy Should Consult Their Healthcare Team, Including Neurologists, Before Starting A New Exercise Program. This Is Especially Important For Those With Uncontrolled Seizures Or Specific Health Concerns.

- **Gradual Introduction:** Starting With Low-Impact And Moderate-Intensity Exercises And Gradually Increasing Intensity And Duration Is Advisable To Minimize Potential Risks.

- **Regular Monitoring:** Individuals With Epilepsy Should Pay Attention To How Their Bodies Respond To Exercise And Be Aware Of Any Potential Triggers. If They Notice An Increase In Seizure Frequency Or Severity, They Should Seek Guidance From Healthcare Professionals.

4. Safety Precautions:

- Buddy System: Exercising With A Partner Or In A Group May Provide An Added Layer Of Safety, Especially For

Those At Risk Of Seizures During Physical Activity.

• **Awareness Of Surroundings:** Individuals With Epilepsy Should Exercise In Safe Environments, Avoiding Activities With A High Risk Of Injury If A Seizure Were To Occur.

5. Medication Adjustments:

• **Medication Management:** The Intensity And Frequency Of Exercise Can Affect The Metabolism Of Antiepileptic Medications. Therefore, Healthcare Professionals May Need To Adjust Medication Dosages To Maintain Therapeutic Levels.

In Summary, While Exercise Has Many Health Benefits, Individuals With

Epilepsy Should Approach It With Caution And Under The Guidance Of Healthcare Professionals. A Personalized Approach, Considering The Individual's Seizure Type, Overall Health, And Potential Triggers, Is Essential. Regular Communication With Healthcare Providers Helps Ensure That Any Exercise Program Is Safe And Aligns With The Specific Needs Of The Individual With Epilepsy.

Conclusion

In Conclusion, The Epilepsy Diet, Particularly The Ketogenic Diet And Its Modifications, Is A Treatment Method That Involves Adjusting Macronutrient Consumption To Manage Epilepsy, Especially In Situations Of Drug-Resistant Seizures. Here Are Crucial Points To Summarize The Information:

1. Dietary Approaches:

• The Ketogenic Diet Is A High-Fat, Low-Carbohydrate, And Moderate-Protein Diet Meant To Produce And Sustain A State Of Ketosis In The Body.

• Variations Include The Modified Atkins Diet (MAD), Medium-Chain

Triglyceride (MCT) Diet, And Low Glycemic Index Treatment (LGIT).

2.   Effectiveness   In   Seizure Management:

• The Epilepsy Diet, Particularly The Ketogenic Diet, Has Proven Success In Reducing Seizure Frequency And Increasing Seizure Control In Some Patients, Especially Those With Drug-Resistant Epilepsy.

3. Mechanisms of Action:

• The Specific Processes By Which The Epilepsy Diet Works Are Not Entirely Understood, But Potential Aspects Include Variations In Metabolism, Stability Of Neuronal Excitability, Neurotransmitter Modulation, Anti-

Inflammatory Effects, Increased Mitochondrial Function, And Epigenetic Changes.

4. Types of Epilepsy Diets:

• Various Types Of Epilepsy Diets, Such As The Conventional Ketogenic Diet, Modified Atkins Diet, MCT Diet, And LGIT, Offer Flexibility Based On Individual Needs And Preferences.

5. Implementation And Considerations:

• Getting Started With The Epilepsy Diet Entails Consultation With Healthcare Specialists, Educational Resources, Meal Planning, Gradual Transition, Monitoring Ketone Levels, And Resolving Potential Obstacles.

6. Foods To Include:

- Include Healthy Fats, Protein Sources, Low-Carbohydrate Veggies, Berries (In Moderation), Herbs And Spices, Low-Glycemic Fruits (In Moderation), Full-Fat Dairy (In Moderation), Beverages Like Water And Herbal Teas, And Nutrient-Dense Foods.

7. Foods To Avoid:

- Avoid High-Carbohydrate Foods, Sugary Foods And Sweeteners, Processed Foods, High-Sugar Fruits, High-Carbohydrate Vegetables, Processed Meats With Added Sugars, Low-Fat Dairy Products, Alcohol, High-

Carbohydrate Sauces, And Certain High-Carbohydrate Nuts And Seeds.

8. Dealing with Side Effects:

• Common Side Effects Of The Epilepsy Diet May Include The "Keto Flu," Digestive Difficulties, Dehydration, Vitamin Deficiencies, Hypoglycemia, Cholesterol Level Fluctuations, Weight Changes, Gastrointestinal Upset, Trouble Adhering To The Diet, And Psychological Impact. Strategies Include Gradual Introduction, Nutritional Changes, Hydration, Electrolyte Supplementation, And Emotional Support.

9. Epilepsy Diet for Different Age Groups:

• The Approach To The Epilepsy Diet Varies For Newborns, Children, Adolescents, Adults, And Seniors. Considerations Include Growth And Development, Lifestyle, Nutritional Demands, And Individual Preferences.

10. Exercise and Impact on Epilepsy:

• Exercise Can Have Both Positive And Complex Impacts On Epilepsy. While It Offers Numerous Health Benefits, Individual Responses May Vary. Precautions And Contact With Healthcare Specialists Are Necessary.

11. Monitoring And Adjusting The Diet:

• Regular Monitoring Encompasses Ketone Testing, Seizure Tracking, Nutritional Assessment, Weight And Growth Monitoring, Gastrointestinal Tolerance Assessment, And Evaluation Of Physical And Mental Well-Being. Adjustments May Be Made Based On Individual Reactions, Medication Management, And Continued Consultation With Healthcare Providers.

To Summarize, The Epilepsy Diet Is A Personalized And Dynamic Approach That Necessitates Meticulous Preparation, Continuous Observation, And Cooperation Among Patients,

Caregivers, And Medical Experts. To Maximize Its Effectiveness In Managing Epilepsy While Taking Into Account Each Person's Particular Needs And Problems, Regular Follow-Up And Changes Are Necessary.

THE END

www.ingramcontent.com/pod-product-compliance
Lightning Source LLC
Chambersburg PA
CBHW061247250726

48653CB00002B/552